T0407341

# The Shrinking Belt

*Crystal's Skinny List to EZ Weight Loss*

Marsha "Crystal" Moore

**BALBOA.**
PRESS
A DIVISION OF HAY HOUSE

Balboa Press books may be ordered through booksellers or by contacting:
Balboa Press
A Division of Hay House
1663 Liberty Drive
Bloomington, IN 47403
www.balboapress.com
1-(877) 407-4847

Author photo by RL Caron, Naples, FL

Printed in the United States of America

ISBN: 978-1-4525-6840-9 (sc)
ISBN: 978-1-4525-6841-6 (e)

Library of Congress Control Number: 2013902524

Balboa Press rev. date: 08/16/2013

# Welcome to *The Shrinking Belt*!

ONE NIGHT WHILE WATCHING TV, I got up to get a glass of water. I returned to my living room and bent down to pet my Shih Tzu, Bentley. When I returned to my recliner, I felt very strange. Had I not known better, I would have sworn that someone had slipped something into the water I drank.

I asked my husband to take my blood pressure. It was an alarming 210/99! The next day I went to see a cardiologist, who not only diagnosed me with high blood pressure but also insisted on a sleep study. And that's how I found out that I really wasn't healthy. Not only did I have high blood pressure but I had sleep apnea.

Both the cardiologist and the sleep doctor told me that if I could lose at least 20-25 pounds, I might be able to lower my blood pressure and avoid using the C-Pap device to keep my airway open while I slept. This was motivation enough for me to begin to re-evaluate what and how I ate. But I knew that I would never make it as a rabbit; a life of nibbling on lettuce and veggies just wasn't going to work. I believed that with a little work I could figure out how to cut empty calories and unnecessary fat from my diet. And so I embarked on a quest to find tasty and satisfying foods at the grocery store that were healthier than my current default choices. So I read labels, made different purchases and taste-tested these new foods. The ones that my taste buds gave "thumbs up" to were added to my grocery list, while the ones that although "healthier" tasted like chemicals, or nothing at all, were ditched. Over time this resulted in a list of new foods that satisfied my palate and helped me reach my goal.

When I lost 30 pounds in 28 weeks, going from a size 14 to a size 6, some of my neighbors thought that I was terminally ill. When they learned that not only was I not ill, but I was healthier than I had been in years, they all wanted to know my secret. I told them my weight loss was due to changing my FAT CALORIE LOADED grocery list to what I had come to call my *SHRINKING BELT* grocery list. Needless to say, those who heard my story wanted a copy of my list, and I gladly shared it. But when friends and neighbors asked if I could make copies for their friends, and then suggested that they would like to *buy* copies of my list to give to others as gifts, I realized that there might be a wider audience who would be interested in what I had learned. So, it can be said that this book was created by popular demand!

Now in the name of full disclosure, let me explain. If you have never heard of me, that's OK because I'm not famous, I'm not a celebrity endorser, and I'm not a weight loss guru. I'm just a regular person who got scared, took control, and as a result, got healthy. I know that some of you who are reading this are in a situation similar to the one I faced. And like me, you're on the go and love to eat. So I say to you, if I did it, so can you! And it will be easier for you than it was for me because I'm sharing my *Shrinking Belt* grocery list with you, as well as other tips that helped me drop the pounds and keep them off. You won't have to spend hours reading labels and buying products that offer less fat but no taste.

When it comes to the foods you love, **what satisfies *you*?** Is it *SPICY, SAUCY, SAVORY, SWEET, CRUNCHY, CHEWY, or SALTY?* The food items on the *Shrinking Belt* list include them all, and they are LOW in calories, LOW in fat, and HIGH in fiber… just what dietitians tell us will help us lose and keep weight off. I have tested each of the products on the *Shrinking Belt* list and I can assure you that there are no cardboard tasting substitutes here! Because I did all the work for you, you can use my list to quickly shop your way to skinny. Simply choose to buy the groceries on this list instead of the ones you would normally buy, eat the portion size listed on the label, and you will melt the fat away and be amazed at **your** *Shrinking Belt.*

Not only will you appreciate the convenience of using the *Shrinking Belt* Shopping list, but I hope you will find my ♥ *Tips* ♥ that are scattered throughout the list, to be helpful in your quest for a healthier life.

To make the shopping experience EZ for you, the *Shrinking Belt* shopping list is presented to you in **categories** that roughly correspond to various aisles found in most grocery stores. As you read the *Shrinking Belt* list, you will notice that at times I list specific brands and at other times I just refer to a more generic product. In some cases this is due to my inability to get permission from the companies whose products I use to list them in this book. At other times, it is because I have found that any number of brands that meet the criteria are interchangeable. It is also important to note that I have received permission to list the product brands without compensation of any kind.

**Important Disclaimer:** Always consult your physician, doctor, or health care provider before beginning any diet, nutrition or exercise program. Those of you that have special dietary needs should be aware that some foods listed in this book may not be appropriate for you.

# Testimonials

Oh my goodness, have your weight loss tips ever helped me! YES!!! From the start I took your tips and implemented them into my lifestyle. It made my weight loss journey much simpler and without sacrifice. From your first tip about the Flatout® and Lavash to your wonderful breakfast waffles, it sure helped me stay focused on my goal, which was to eat healthier. Your own weight loss journey was/is such an inspiration to me. The excitement in your voice when you shared a new weight loss tip was infectious and helped me stay on track. Thank you Crystal for your encouragement and continuous enthusiasm as we win the battle of the bulge! Hugs...

Bonnie Clark, Estero, Florida

Simplicity is Crystal Moore's brilliance! I have never seen anyone lose weight and keep it off as effortlessly and elegantly as she has.

Pepi Palmer, Bonita Springs, Florida

# FINALLY, A NO BRAINER SOLUTION TO LOSING WEIGHT!

M.O.M, FLORIDA

Your weight loss tips were the answer to a dieter's dream. Without them I do not believe I could have lost as much weight as I did and certainly not as quickly. By incorporating your tips in my meals, I saved calories and the meals were much more palatable. They increased my enjoyment of my meals and I looked forward to the menus. You taught me that a diet was not about what I could not have but what I *could* have. The change in attitude made a huge difference. But as I watched you lose weight a year ahead of me, you gave me the incentive to finally take the step. I have passed much of your information on to others facing the challenge of a diet and they have all been very grateful for the tips. Your upbeat personality is a blessing I would not want to have missed.

SUSAN, ELKHART, INDIANA

Crystal has done the legwork on helping you make good choices at the grocery store!

NANCY, PLANTATION, FLORIDA

What a great idea! This little book has saved me so much time. It has truly been a lifesaver. I run a busy schedule always coming and going in a hurry. This little booklet stays in my purse. When I need to dash to the store I am always prepared. I recently started my "change of lifestyle" eating habits. Going to the store used to be time consuming and frustrating. Not knowing what I was supposed to eat and where to find it was causing me to make bad choices. Having Crystal's book changed that. It was all there in an easy to read little book. Her book is full of easy concoctions and ideas that keeps me eating healthy foods. I don't leave home without it! Being able to lose weight has been something I have struggled with pretty much my adult life. I have been successful in losing 25 pounds and managing the weight loss to date, thanks to Crystal's book. It is truly empowering!

DANA, NAPLES, FLORIDA

Now, get ready to CINCH YOUR BELT!
Enjoy quick and EZ shopping, and delicious meals.
Buy the right foods and watch
the pounds melt away!!!

Let's get *Crystal* Clear:

**Portion control is very important.** Always ask yourself if you are satisfied *before* you finish your meal. Be honest and you'll soon see that the second portion you think you want will actually be another meal for you…like a 2-for-1 meal or a BOGO (buy one get one free)!

**Change all of your food choices to the following:**

| | |
|---|---|
| LOW FAT | SUGAR FREE |
| REDUCED FAT | LOW SUGAR |
| FAT FREE | NO SUGAR ADDED |
| LOW SODIUM | LOW CALORIE |

Now get ready to CINCH YOUR BELT! Enjoy quick and EZ shopping and delicious meals. Buy the right foods, eat the right portions, and watch the pounds melt away!!!

## Baking and Nuts

### Carnation® Fat Free Evaporated Milk

♥ *Use in baking, coffee* ♥

### Shredded Coconut Reduced Fat

(May not be in your grocery store, but usually can be found in a health food store)

♥ *Sprinkle on hot (yummy on oatmeal) or cold cereal, fruit salad* ♥

♥ *Roll a banana in coconut and freeze for a lip-smacking snack* ♥

### Baked Goods Mixes

Krusteaz® Fat Free Cranberry-Orange Muffin Mix
Krusteaz® Blueberry Muffin Mix
Krusteaz® Fat Free Fudge Brownie Mix

♥ *These low-fat baked goods will satisfy your sweet tooth and are so good that family and guests will rave about them. Be careful to limit yourself to the recommended portions* ♥

### Olive Oil, Olive Oil Spray or other non-stick spray

♥ *Substitute olive oil for other oils in cooking and use 1 tablespoon with lemon juice or vinegar to use in salads or for dipping* ♥

## NUTS

Almonds

♥ *One of the most nutritious nuts; an excellent source of protein with no cholesterol. Try finely ground as a coating for fish, chicken and meats* ♥

Pecans

♥ *Add "wow" to a waffle by adding some sliced banana, drizzling on some sugar-free maple syrup, sprinkling on chopped pecans and topping it all with fat-free whipped cream!* ♥

Peanuts, dry-roasted with sea salt

♥ *Great as a snack when you just have to have something salty! But watch the portion* ♥

Pumpkin Seeds

Walnuts

Soy Nuts

♥ *A great combo with dried cranberries added to a salad* ♥

"Lose weight slowly with small changes."

## Syrup

Sugar-free maple syrup

Sugar-free chocolate syrup

♥ *Less messy than the powdered and EZ to pour in coffee and onto frozen treats* ♥

## Breading

Corn Meal

100% whole wheat bread crumbs

Ground almonds

Panko Bread Crumbs

♥ *Try making mocked fried chicken by lightly spraying chicken tenders with olive oil and then rolling in one of these breadings. Bake on cookie sheet in a 350 degree oven* ♥

## Extracts

Almond

Mint

Vanilla

♥ *Great for flavoring coffee/teas and baking* ♥

## Spices - a variety

Cinnamon

Crushed Red Pepper & Cayenne Pepper (Puts the zip in your do-dah!)

Garlic – chopped or powder

Lemon Pepper seasoning

Mustard (dry)

Pumpkin Spice

Salt - Sea Salt and salt-free seasonings

♥ *These are my favorite spices, but all spices are OK. But be sure to check spice blends for hidden sugar and sodium* ♥

## BUTTER SUBSTITUTE

Butter Buds® Sprinkles All Natural Butter Flavor Granules

♥ *Sprinkle on potatoes, popcorn, vegetables* ♥

♥ *Dissolve in warm water, add a dash of garlic salt or minced garlic, and you have the perfect dipping sauce for lobster, crab or shrimp* ♥

## SUGAR SUBSTITUTE

♥ *There are many brands of sugar substitutes but the best ones will say either Stevia or Xylitol* ♥

## CONDIMENTS

Bacon Bits or Bacon pieces

♥ *Look for reduced fat and reduced sodium* ♥

## BBQ Sauce

Walden Farms® Bar-B-Q Sauce

♥ *No fat, no salt, no sugar Zippy topping for all meats and fish* ♥

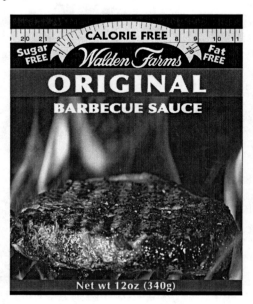

## Crouton Substitutes

Fresh Gourmet® Tri-Colored Tortilla Strips and Santa Fe Tortilla Strips

Fresh Gourmet® Crispy Onions

♥ *"Crunchies" are a necessity! Keep these in stock at all times to add to salads, soups, sandwiches, wraps and for dining out* ♥

## KETCHUP

Walden Farms® or other reduced-sugar ketchup

## MAYONNAISE

Smart Balance® Light Mayonnaise Dressing

Smart Beat® Nonfat Mayonnaise Dressing.

## MUSTARD

❤ *Any kind you want. Just make sure there is no sugar added, so best to avoid sweet mustards* ❤

## OLIVES

## CAPERS

## JALAPENOS

## PICKLES AND RELISH

Mt. Olive No Sugar Sweet Gherkins

Mt. Olive No Sugar Bread & Butter Spears

Mt. Olive No Sugar Bread & Butter Chips

Mt. Olive No Sugar Bread & Butter Sandwich Stuffers

Mt. Olive No Sugar Relish

"Stay active and focus on you!"

## Salad Dressings

Walden Farms® Fat Free

♥ *Any fat-free dressing is OK* ♥

## Salsas/Hot Sauce

♥ *For those of us who like "Zip in our Do-Dah" there is nothing like sauces to spice up our food. But not all sauces are created equal. Some have sugar added, others are needlessly full of sodium/salt. When buying your favorite sauce, choose only low sodium and be sure there is no sugar added* ♥

## Low Sodium Soy Sauce/Teriyaki Sauce

### Beverages

## Alcohol Beverages

Lite Beer

Lite Vodka

Lite Margarita

♥ *When it comes to comparing calories, you can enjoy 12 oz. of LITE BEER vs. 4 oz. of wine or other spirits* ♥

## Coffee

♥ *Use sugar-free creamers. REDUCED FAT EGGNOG is great as a coffee creamer* ♥

## Juices

V8® Low Sodium Juice

♥ *Add to homemade or canned soups to either thin or enhance flavor* ♥

V8 Diet Splash® - **ZESTY!**

## FRUIT JUICES

♥ *Look for No Sugar Added, Low Sodium, Low calorie. Diet Cranberry, or Lite Cranberry is my fave!* ♥

## SUGAR-FREE POWDERED DRINK MIXES

♥ *There are a variety of flavors to please everyone and features to-go packs to add to bottled water* ♥

## SODAS

Diet Sodas *without* sodium, such as lemon-lime, orange, and cola

Sugar-free Diet Tonic

Seltzer.

## TEA

Green Tea

Black Tea

Herbal Tea

## WATER

♥ *Flavored water is refreshing but has some calories. Watch the sodium and sugar! Make your own by adding the rind of an entire lemon or orange to a pitcher of water* ♥

## BREAD PRODUCTS

### BAGELS

Thomas® Bagel Thins™ 100% Whole Wheat

♥ *Spread on some Fat-Free cream cheese, add smoked salmon (lox), diced red onions and capers – delicious!* ♥

Reduced Fat Whole Wheat Biscuits

### BREAD

Merita® LITE Whole Wheat

Pepperidge Farm® Light-Style Bread Extra Fiber - 40 calories per slice!

### BUNS (BURGER/HOT DOG)

Merita® LITE Whole Wheat Hamburger Buns

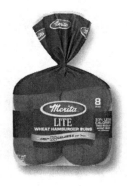

Merita® LITE Whole Wheat Hot Dog Buns

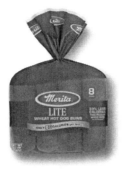

♥ *They're the best. EAT WITHOUT GUILT!!!* ♥

## CRACKERS

Flatout® Edge On™

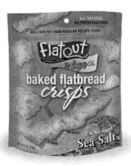

Pepperidge Farm® Baked Naturals™

> "Cut your food in small pieces, use a smaller plate and eat slowly."

## Flatbread

Flatout® Flatbread Healthy Grain

Flatout® Flatbread Light Spinach

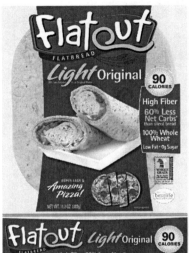
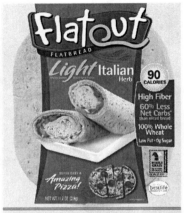
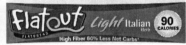

♥ *Great bread and cracker substitutes that save on calories. Use as a tasty base for quiche, Low Fat/Low Calorie pizza crust and wraps* ♥

## Lavash

♥ *A delicious, wholesome flatbread usually found in health food stores* ♥

## Muffins

Thomas® Better Start™ Light multi-grain English Muffins

## TORTILLAS

La Tortilla Factory® Smart and Delicious™ Whole Wheat and Soft Wraps™

La Tortilla Factory® Whole Grain Rye with Olive Oil

La Tortilla Factory® Whole Wheat Low-Carb High Fiber.

♥ *They also have a unique blend of corn and wheat* ♥

Tam-X-icos® Corn Tortillas

Tam-X-icos® Whole Wheat Lo-Carb

♥ *All are yummy! Located in the refrigerated cooler section* ♥

## CANNED FOODS

### ARTICHOKES

♥ *Choose oil-free brands packed in <u>water</u>. Great in pasta salads!* ♥

### BEANS

Bush's Best® Grillin' Beans® Black Bean Fiesta

♥ *Adds a new twist on non-chili dogs! Use as a zesty salsa. Load in a wrap* ♥

Plain Beans

♥ *Buy low-sodium beans; drain and rinse. Beans are so versatile, filling and loaded with fiber* ♥

## Chili Beans

Joan of Arc Chili®

- ♥ *For a meatless meal, add onions, reduced-fat cheeses and top with Fresh Gourmet® Crispy Onions* ♥

## Refried Beans

- ♥ *Look for Fat Free. A must for nachos or a layered Mexican dip* ♥

## Turkey

## Chicken

## Fish

- ♥ *Salmon and tuna packed in <u>water</u>. Clams added to pasta add extra chewing* ♥

## Fruit – No Sugar Added

## Pumpkin (Pie Filling) – see Crystal's Concoctions

## Sauerkraut

- ♥ *Load this on sandwiches, hot dogs or wraps* ♥

## Vegetables – Always look for Low-Sodium varieties.

## CEREALS

Post® Shredded Wheat

Post® Shredded Wheat 'n Bran

Oatmeal – UNSWEETENED

♥ *Add chopped apples, cinnamon, and drizzle with Sugar-Free maple syrup* ♥

## DAIRY

Butter/Margarine - Choose Light or olive oil spreads.

Smart Beat® Fat Free Squeeze Margarine

## CHEESES

♥ *Opt for Fat-Free or Low-Fat feta, mozzarella, cheddar, cream cheese and cottage cheese* ♥

## LIGHT CHEESE WEDGES - AN ARRAY OF DELICIOUS FLAVORS

## REDUCED-FAT CHEESE

Reduced Fat Parmesan

Cabot® Reduced Fat Cheese

"Never crash diet or your diet will crash."

**\*Reduced-Fat cheeses are better for melts!** (Fat-free cheeses are "rubbery" when melted.)

♥ *A variety of reduced-fat cheeses makes a great cheese platter…Perfect for entertaining* ♥

## Yogurt

Dannon Light & Fit® Yogurt

Dannon Light & Fit® Greek Yogurt

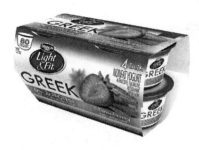

♥ *Great on waffles for that saucy taste!* ♥

## Hannah Tzatziki Greek Style Cucumber & Garlic Yogurt Dip

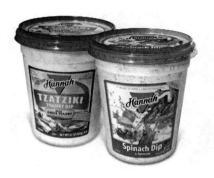

## EGGS OR EGG SUBSTITUTE

## MILK

Choose Skim/Non-Fat only. Dry Fat-Free versions are fine.

♥ *Add Sugar-Free Chocolate Syrup for tasty chocolate milk* ♥

## SOUR CREAM - FAT FREE OR LOW FAT

## FAT-FREE WHIPPED CREAM

♥ *Another must-have! Great to top off waffles, pumpkin pie, ice cream and frozen yogurt…. even in your coffee!* ♥

## DESSERTS

Pumpkin Pie - Check out Crystal's Concoctions

Fat-Free or Sugar-Free puddings – add a dollop of Fat-Free whipped cream.

Angel Food Cake

## DESSERTS - FROZEN

EDY's® Fat-Free Frozen Yogurt Blends™

Reduced-Fat Cheesecake

"Eat socially, not liberally."

## WAFFLES

Van's Natural Foods™ Lite Waffles - whole-grains with a touch of cinnamon.

♥ *This makes a great base for pumpkin pie or strawberry shortcake* ♥

## FREEZER SECTION FAVORITES

## BURGERS - MEATLESS, TURKEY, SALMON, GROUPER, MAHI MAHI

## KAHIKI® EGG ROLLS

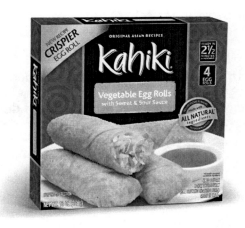

♥ *Substitute the sugary sauce provided. Mix a small amount of Chinese mustard and ketchup for dipping* ♥

## LEAN CUISINE® ENTREES

♥ *Look for meals with whole wheat pasta, brown rice or multigrain!* ♥

## LEAN POCKETS® VARIETY WITH WHOLE WHEAT

## COOKED CHICKEN STRIPS, (GRILLED)

♥ *Ideal for a quick meal, salads, soup and wraps* ♥

## GROUND TURKEY

♥ *For meat loaves, casseroles, spaghetti sauce, tacos* ♥

## CELENTANO® TURKEY MEATBALLS

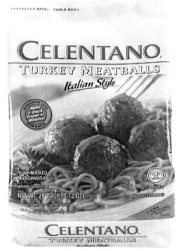

♥ *Serve as appetizers, or use in sauces and soups* ♥

"Stay focused on being healthy,
not on becoming thin."

## Shrimp and Scallops

## Shaw's Premier Seafood™ Key West Style Grouper Burgers and Lump Crab Cakes

♥ *Top with mango salsa…mmm!* ♥

## Trident Seafoods® Pacific Salmon Burgers

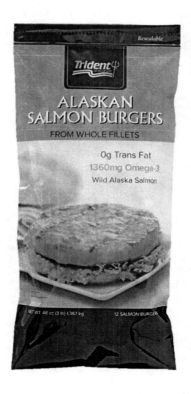

♥ *Slice into a Flatout® wrap with dry coleslaw, fat-free feta cheese and Tzatziki dip…marvelous!!!* ♥

# Trident Seafoods® Wild Mahi Mahi Burgers...*ALOHA!!!*

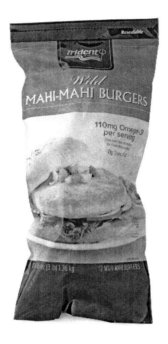

## Fruits

♥ *I love berries and melon. Great for quick smoothies!* ♥

## Veggies (without the buttery sauce)

♥ *Add thawed chopped spinach to soups, Tzatziki dip, sour cream or omelets. Just drain, rinse and add* ♥

## Pepper Stir Fry

♥ *A colorful and versatile addition to most recipes* ♥

## FRUITS (FRESH)

### APPLES

♥ *Deliciously crunchy on salads with your favorite cheese crumbles; a great snack or appetizer* ♥

### BANANAS

♥ *A natural, healthy sweet.* **Check out Crystal's Concoctions!** ♥

### LEMONS AND LIMES

♥ *Flavor water, sauces, add a squeeze of lime to your beer...aah!* ♥

### PAPAYAS AND MELONS

♥ *Cut in half and add a scoop of shrimp or chicken salad. Add to a leafy green salad for a surprising zest!* ♥

### GRAPES AND BLUEBERRIES

♥ *Freeze for healthy snacking...nature's candy!* ♥

## JAMS, PRESERVES AND PEANUT BUTTER

Polaner® Sugar Free with Fiber Preserves and Marmalade

Smart Balance® Rich Roast Chunky Peanut Butter

"Exercise for sustained weight loss."

# Lean Meats and Fish

## Canadian Bacon

## Hot Dogs

♥ *Fat-Free Turkey, Fat-Free Smoked White Turkey or Fat-Free Chicken are the best…I am hooked!!!* ♥

## Fish

Salmon, scallops, shrimp, grouper, tilapia, tuna and mahi-mahi are my ultimate favorites!

♥ *Top with mango salsa and you're ready to dance!* ♥

## Meats

♥ *Opt for skinless chicken, turkey and lean pork. If you choose beef, look for lean cuts* ♥

## Pizza Topping

♥ *Turkey Pepperoni or Lean Italian Turkey Sausage are delicious. Italian Turkey Sausage is also great for breakfast* ♥

## Sandwich Meats

♥ *Choose low sodium and low fat* ♥

## Sausage

Reduced-Fat Sausages or Reduced Fat-Kielbasa

Breakfast sausages - Lite

# <u>Munchies</u>

## Salty Snacks

**Popcorn** - Jolly Time® Healthy Pop®

♥ *This popcorn has more chews per kernel than other leading brands. Eat one piece at a time* ♥

Any 94% fat-free popcorn

## Potato Chips

Baked, Light or Reduced Fat

♥ *Buy the crinkled variety…adds more Crunch* ♥

## Snikiddy® all natural Baked Fries…A MUST

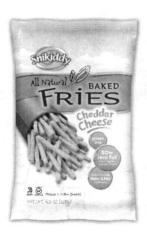 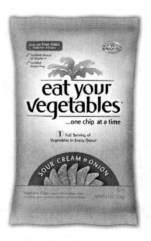

♥ *Want More Crunch Time??? Break the chips in half or thirds and crunch slowly* ♥

## <u>SWEET SNACKS</u>

### BROTHERS ALL-NATURAL™ FRUIT CRISPS

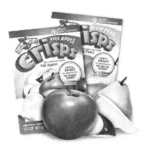

♥ *Freeze-Dried fruit makes a healthy snack; super EZ and packable for long travel. Munch with sandwiches instead of chips. Stores like Costco offer big, cost-saving packages that last. Eat with a glass of water before a meal; curbs appetite* ♥

### DARK CHOCOLATE WITH AT LEAST 70% COCOA

♥ *1 oz. semi-sweet satisfies your sweet tooth* ♥

### FRUIT DIPPED IN WALDEN FARMS® CALORIE FREE CHOCOLATE DIP

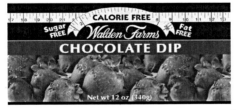

♥ *Check out* **Crystal's Concoctions** *for frozen chocolate banana* ♥

### SUGAR-FREE CANDY

## Pastas and Grains
**\*\*If allergic to whole wheat, buy
Gluten-Free products.\*\***

### Barley

♥ *Adds ROBUST without the BUST! Add to soups or serve as a side dish* ♥

### Hodgson Mill® 100% Whole Wheat, Whole Grain Pasta

♥ *Provide the most variety of pastas* ♥

\*Remember: Look for the words*"100% Whole Wheat"* (not BLEND).

### Seeds of Change®

♥ *Delicious variety of pre-cooked grains that are quick and EZ to microwave.* **Quinoa and Whole Grain Brown Rice** *are the best* ♥

### Quinoa (pronounced *keen-wa*)

♥ *Quinoa is a healthier substitute for bread stuffing, or use as a side dish. It's a great base for stir fry* ♥

### Rice

Brown Rice

Wild Rice

---

"A pedometer is your best accessory."

## FLAX SEED

♥ *Mega Benefits! It contains Omega-3, Protein and Fiber. Add to waffles, tuna or chicken salad, cereals or yogurt* ♥

## SAUCES AND GRAVY

## ALFREDO SAUCE

Buitoni® Light Alfredo Sauce

♥ *Located in refrigerated section near cheeses and prepared pasta* ♥

## CREAM SAUCES

Campbell's® Healthy Request® Cream of Mushroom soup, Cream of Celery soup, Cream of Chicken soup - 98% Fat Free.

♥ *Makes great sauces, gravy, and low-fat Alfredo sauce* ♥

## GRAVY

Franco-American® Slow Roast® 99% Fat-Free Turkey or Chicken Gravy

"Put on some great music and dance around the house while doing your chores."

## Pasta Sauce

Francesco Rinaldi® TO BE
HEALTHY® with Omega 3

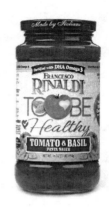

♥ *Try all varieties. No need to
add spices. Mangiamo!!!* ♥

## Other brands

Look for the words "No Sugar
Added" or "Light."

♥ *I add Italian spices to enhance
the flavor* ♥

## Pesto Sauce

Available in a jar or package

## <u>Soups</u>

Campbell's® Select Harvest® Light

♥ *Select the variety that includes whole wheat pasta
and whole grains* ♥

## Chicken Broth

♥ *Choose 100% fat free and at least 33% less sodium
than regular broth* ♥

"Call a friend instead of reaching
for the wrong food."

## <u>VEGETABLES (FRESH) -</u><br><u>EAT AS MUCH AS YOU WANT!</u>

Avocados, Broccoli, Brussels sprouts, and Bell Peppers

## DRY COLESLAW MIX – A MUST

- ♥ *Use in salads, sandwiches, wraps. It's less costly than lettuce, stays fresh longer, and gives plenty of CRUNCH! This is a Crystal's staple* ♥

## CARROTS

- ♥ *Opt for the crinkle cut variety; stays fresh and juicy longer than baby carrots* ♥

## GARLIC - FRESH, DRIED, POWDERED

## MUSHROOMS AND ONIONS

## POTATOES

Small/medium

- ♥ *Great baked and topped with Tzatziki dip or Fat-Free sour cream, Low-Sodium bacon bits and crispy onions. Best to limit one per day…No Fries!* ♥

"Don't save your larger clothes; donate to a thrift shop."

## Tomatoes

Cherry or grape tomatoes

♥ *Great for snacking as well as in salads* ♥

Sun-dried tomatoes packaged without olive oil

♥ *Use in omelets, pizza topping, leafy salads, wraps, sandwiches, pasta and rice salads and casseroles* ♥

## Spinach

♥ *Cover your plate with this super food and place your entrée on top. Also a perfect substitute for lettuce. Include spinach in your sandwiches* ♥

## Sweet Potatoes

♥ *Healthier than white potatoes and naturally sweet* ♥

## Zucchini/Yellow Squash

♥ *Use slices as a healthy base for appetizers or add to salads, soups and pasta* ♥

"Keep this book in your purse at all times."

## "MOORE" WEIGHT LOSS TIPS FOR DINING OUT

WHEN PLACING YOUR ORDER ASK for a take-home container and place half of your meal in it to avoid over-eating.

### LOOKING AT THE MENU:

Say **NO, NO, NO** to fried, battered, breaded, crispy, creamy or buttery sauces such as Scalloped, Au gratin. Hollandaise, Scampi.

**Say YES to: baked, boiled, broiled, grilled, poached, roasted, steamed, without butter** (bring your own **Butter Buds)**

Ask for Low-Fat or Fat-Free salad dressings (on the side).

Take a bag of toasted "crunchies" such as **Fresh Gourmet® tortilla strips** to top an omelet, salad or soup. They're a great substitute for the fried, salty tortilla chips at Mexican restaurants. Or take low-carb whole wheat or corn tortillas with you. The waiters don't care! If you forget to plan ahead, order the corn tortillas for dipping or as a soft taco/burrito. **Huge Difference on your scale the next morning!**

Know which Italian restaurants use 100% whole wheat pastas, pizza crusts or breads, and dine at those places only.

When ordering a meal with sauces, request pesto sauce or marinara instead of creamy sauces.

Check Websites or call them to verify your selected choices, and keep your list handy.

**Breakfast** - Take a small container with Fat-Free cream cheese and **Polaner® Sugar Free with Fiber Preserves** to spread on dry whole wheat toast. Omelets are usually too much for one person. For two people, split a bowl of fruit and the omelet. It's best to eat the fruit first.

**Lunch** - Hungry for a Reuben? Take a small container of Fat-Free 1000 Island dressing and a bag of crunchies (Fresh Gourmet®). Ask for dry whole wheat toast, a blackened fish fillet, (or turkey), extra sauerkraut and Swiss cheese (optional). I always remove the second slice of bread and combine the fish or turkey onto one slice, creating an open-face Reuben topped with crunchies. Ask for the dressing on the side. Extremely satisfying!

**Salad Bars** - Fill up on the fresh vegetables items and use the Fat-Free dressings. The prepared salads tend to have more of what we *don't need!* If you're not satisfied, have just a TASTE of the prepared salads.

**Pizza Night** - take toasted flatbread with you and transfer the pizza toppings onto your flatbread. You'll see that 1 flatbread will hold toppings from 2 pizza slices, without the extra calories. If you forget your toasted flatbread, order the thin crust, and place 2 toppings on 1 slice. Always use a fork and knife to eat pizza, as you'll feel satisfied sooner than eating it with your hands.

**Seafood Sensations** - Take a small container **of Butter Buds®,** a MUST when having seafood, especially *Lobster.* Ask for a ½ cup of very hot water and add a splash of olive oil, stir in **Butter Buds®.** ENJOY and LOSE THE POUNDS!

Sprinkle fresh lemon juice and some Butter Buds® on top of all of your vegetables before cooking or when dining out. Add to mashed potatoes instead of butter or margarine.

*When eating fish*:

A small container of **Hannah Tzatziki Dip** with **Mt Olive No Sugar Added Sweet Relish,** and a dash of lemon juice easily replaces tartar sauce. **Walden Farms® Seafood Sauce** replaces the high-calorie/high-sugar regular Seafood Sauce.

**Bread -** No "KNEAD" to say NO to bread - When a basket of bread is placed in front of you, ask for olive oil and parmesan cheese. Hollow out the bread and dip pieces of the crust in the oil and cheese… instant satisfaction without guilt!

## "Moore" Hints for Happy Hour ☺

Limit wine and cocktails and switch to a LITE BEER.

When drinking wine, fill the glass with lots of ice. (I do the same with my beer mug.) You drink less and it's less potent.

Instead of a Bloody Mary, have a Bloody Mary Jane – vegetable juice with vodka. It'll curb your appetite before dinner. Vodka Lite does exist!

Finally, a Margarita Lite! Liquor stores now carry a variety of reduced-calorie drinks.

A few ounces of liquor with seltzer, diet tonic or sodium-free diet soda is OK. You know your limits!

## "Moore" Tips for Entertaining

### Potlucks

Choose to bring at least 3 low-fat dishes or appetizers and eat only the ones you brought if everything else is fattening!

If you're the hostess and guests will be bringing a dish…specify a Low-Fat appetizer, entrée or dessert.

## CRYSTAL'S TASTY CONCOCTIONS

**Remember:**
- ♥ *The appearance of your meal should be as colorful as possible!*
- ♥ *Texture is very important!*
- ♥ *Portion control is extremely important!*
- ♥ *Ask yourself if you are satisfied…don't wait till you're full to ask!!!*

**Asian Soup** – Use Fat-Free and Low-Sodium chicken broth, dry coleslaw mix, stir fry vegetables with Low-Sodium soy sauce - more bulk and no fat! Add left over lean meats/chicken for a heartier meal.

**C' Moore's "Cinchy" Cheeseball/Holiday Losing Log** - Fat-Free Cream Cheese, Low-Fat shredded cheese, add your favorites ingredients:

- ♥ *Sun dried tomatoes, garlic, Italian spices*
- ♥ *Dried fruit and nuts*

Place on wax paper- roll ball or log on sesame seeds, chopped almonds, or other nuts.

Spread on Flatout® Edge On™ Baked Flatbread Crisps.

Bring this fabulous appetizer to all your gatherings, so you are in control to enjoy!

**C' Moore's Egg Muffin Melt** - spray non-stick oil in a small, shallow bowl; place a slice of turkey ham or Canadian Bacon in bowl, pour in a small amount of southwestern style egg substitute and microwave until done. Sprinkle with reduced-fat shredded cheese and place on a toasted Lite Whole Wheat English Muffin.

**Coffee** - For diet friendly and delicious "café mocha," add sugar-free chocolate syrup or a half of a package of fat-free hot chocolate to your coffee with a few dashes of cinnamon and microwave until hot. Top with fat-free whipped cream – mmm!

♥ *For Holidays (or anytime you want to treat yourself) use Reduced-Fat or Lite Eggnog as a creamer and add a dash of nutmeg. Great taste with less calories!*

**Coleslaw** – Add to dry coleslaw: chopped apples, pineapple or mangos for a refreshing zing!

Use in wraps and sandwiches for bulk and fiber without the fat. For dressing use low-fat or fat-free mayonnaise or Tzatziki yogurt dip.

**Cranberry Sauce (Homemade)** Follow the directions on the bag and use a sugar substitute.

Make a large batch and freeze in small containers. Smear your wrap or bread with low-fat or fat-free cream cheese, add turkey or chicken, top with cranberry sauce. It is *Berrylicious!!!*

Note: at this time no one has created a reduced-sugar or no-sugar-added Cranberry Sauce.

**Flatbread Wraps – Awesome Appetizers**
Cut flatbread into rectangular shapes with a pizza cutter, add shrimp and Tzatziki dip and wrap.

Cut into triangles, and toast or bake until crisp. Make extra and put them in small bags for quick, on-the-go munchies. To enhance the flavor, drizzle some of your favorite fat-free salad dressing on them before baking!

Un-toasted flatbread replaces the crust for your Low-Fat quiche (also use an egg substitute for the filling.) Flatbreads can also be grilled like a Panini sandwich or a grilled cheese sandwich, reducing the calories.

**Frozen Desserts** – For a **Skinny Banana Split**, use **Edy's® Fat Free Yogurt Blends** (Frozen Yogurt)**, Polaner® Sugar Free with Fiber Preserves** (try apricot, strawberry, raspberry or orange marmalade), top with fat-free whipped cream and a fresh cherry…Yummy!

**Frozen Chocolate-Covered Bananas** are EZ! Place **Walden Farms® Sugar Free Chocolate Dip** lengthwise on wax paper, with a banana laid lengthwise on one side and a layer of chopped nuts on the other side. Roll the banana in the chocolate to cover and then onto the nuts. Lift the wax paper, place banana in a rectangular plastic container and freeze.

**Hot Dogs** - Add to **Joan of Arc® Chili** or **Bush's Best® Grillin' Beans® Black Bean Fiesta** and microwave until hot; top with diced onions and Fat-Free cheese. Try 2 hot dogs on 1 toasted **Merita®** Lite Wheat Hot Dog Bun with mustard, lots of sauerkraut and topped with **Fresh Gourmet® Crispy Onions**. Or, slice and lightly brown hot dog and add to scrambled eggs (egg substitute). Less fat and calories than regular light turkey sausages! Very satisfying and filling!

For appetizers: cut each dog into six, 1-inch pieces and marinade with Walden Farms® BBQ Sauce. Hot or Cold, Very Tasty!!!

**PASTA** - pasta salad is wonderful cold or heated. After cooking and cooling, toss tube or spiral pasta with your favorite marinade or sauce *before* adding other ingredients for *maximum flavor within each bite!* Add high-fiber vegetables like artichokes and broccoli, and sun-dried tomatoes. **Hodgson Mill®** pastas are my faves! **Francesco Rinaldi® To Be Healthy is the Ultimate Sauce!**

**Pumpkin Pie (No Crust)** Follow the directions on the can of pumpkin, using an egg substitute, Fat-Free evaporated milk, and sugar replacement. Spray the bottom and sides of the pan with a non-stick cooking spray. Use a toasted Low-Fat waffle as the base.

With or without a waffle base, line the pan with chopped almonds. Add the filling and bake. When ready to serve, top it off with Fat-Free whipped cream. *My husband likes to add Fat-Free frozen vanilla yogurt on top of the pumpkin, then add Fat-Free whipped cream...a blast to his craving!

**Salad** – To fresh spinach or lettuce, add Fat-Free walnut oil and raspberry vinaigrette, soy nuts, dried cranberries and Fat-Free Feta Cheese. WOW! Add your favorite fruit and nuts to leafy greens!

**Soft Tortillas or Wraps – La Tortilla Factory® Smart & Delicious™ Tortillas, and Soft Wraps™** Toast or bake for nachos and tostadas. Heat for soft tacos, burritos, or enchiladas. Grill for quesadillas or use as a substitute for a low-cal Panini or grilled sandwiches.

**Tam-X-icos® Corn tortillas -** are excellent in replacing pasta for a tamale pie (*Mexican Lasagna*) and casserole dishes. Use with **Bush's Best® Grillin' Beans® Black Bean Fiesta** and *reduced-fat cheese* alternating with layers, and bake till heated.

Use a pizza cutter and cut into 1/8's, then bake or toast. Store them in a tightly sealed container and take them along when dining out or as nighttime munchies with salsa.

**Stir-Fry Veggies Frozen or Fresh** – Makes a tasty stir-fry with leftover cooked lean meats, Low-Sodium teriyaki sauce and slivered or sliced almonds. Or add your favorite salad dressing and your favorite Low-Fat crumbled cheese.

**Frozen or Fresh Pepper Stir Fry** - chop into omelets, pasta salads, soups and dips.

**Sweet Potatoes** - These are great cooked and mashed with Sugar-Free maple syrup and topped with chopped pecans. Or, slice and spray with olive oil, top with chopped nuts and bake until done.

**Hannah Spinach Dip-already prepared!**
A great spread for wraps and sandwiches. Try it as a replacement for tartar sauce. Delicious topping for Salmon Burgers!

**Hannah Tzatziki Dip** - I use this wonderful and **versatile** dip in place of sour cream, mayonnaise, and even as a seafood cocktail sauce!

♥ *Try Tzatziki with chopped spinach for a delectable spinach dip, then use it as a topping on a baked potato. Spread it on wraps!*

♥ *Add Tzatziki dip to mashed avocado for a great Greek Guacamole dip! Spread on sandwiches or wraps.*

♥ *Add it to dry coleslaw mix for use in wraps or chicken, tuna, or seafood salad.*

♥ *For Tartar Sauce - Add* **Mt. Olive No Sugar Added Sweet Relish**

**Waffles – Van's Natural Foods™ Lite** For a "U DESERVIT" breakfast, add Fat-Free frozen vanilla yogurt and top with lightly simmered chopped apples, cinnamon and some chopped nuts!

For dessert, top with sliced banana and blueberries, a drizzle of Sugar-Free maple syrup, add chopped pecans and Fat-Free whipped cream – perfect! Sprinkle with Flax Seed (optional).

For a cool treat, take a 4 oz. cup Key Lime Pie Yogurt and mix with ½ cup or scoop of Fat-Free vanilla frozen yogurt in a small bowl, and re-freeze for 35-40 min. Use a fork/ knife to gently break mixture away from the edge, turn the bowl upside-down onto a toasted waffle. Top with your favorite crunchy cereal. Get creative with other flavor yogurts and add fruits, like a mashed banana and berries. Wow! That will start your day off with enthusiasm!

Now that you're off to a great start, experiment and share your own creative concoctions with me by going to www.theshrinkingbelt.com. Can't wait to hear from you!!

# Special Request Order Form

Customer Printed Name:             Date Ordered

Phone:

E-Mail address:

Please continue to order and keep in stock the following!

Brand Name Item Quantity

    1.

    2.

    3.

    4.

    5.

    6.

    7.

Thank you for placing my order!

# Crystal's Costco List

***For those of you that think buying in bulk is too much for your household…SHARE with friends and family… SHARE the cost! You will save $$$ and Shrink the Belt!

### CANNED GOODS

Kirkland Signature™ Green Beans with Sea Salt
Mushrooms
Black Beans
Diced Tomatoes
Kirkland Signature™ Albacore Tuna packed in water
Salmon

### SPICES

Kirkland Signature™ Organic Olive oil
Kirkland Signature™ Spices-No-Salt Seasoning
Fresh Gourmet® Crispy Onions

### GRAINS

Flax Seed
Quinoa
Almonds
Seeds of Change® Quinoa and Brown Rice

### PRESERVES

Polaner® Sugar-Free with Fiber Preserves
Dried Fruit

## CHIPS

Brothers-All-Natural™ Fruit Crisps
Snikiddy® all natural Baked Fries

## BREADS

La Tortilla Factory® Smart & Delicious™ Wraps
   and Tortillas
Flat Out® Flat Bread Wraps

## REFRIGERATED ITEMS

Hannah Tzatziki Yogurt Dip
Hannah Spinach Dip
Mango Salsa
Stuffed Grape Leaves
Finlandia® reduced-fat cheese slices (Variety of 4 cheeses)
Dannon® Light & Fit® Yogurt
Fruits and Vegetables
V8® Juice Low Sodium
Chicken, lean pork, turkey

## FROZEN FOODS

Trident Seafoods® Pacific Salmon Burgers
Wild Mahi-Mahi Burgers
Kirkland Signature™ Panko Shrimp
Kirkland Signature™ Wild Alaskan Cod
Fish or Seafood
Lean Cuisine® and Lean Pockets®

## <u>OUT OF THE OVEN</u>

Can't leave without Costco's famous Rotisserie Chicken

**This list was formulated solely by Crystal Moore for your convenience. The Costco products listed are subject to change and may vary by region.

*** THE FINAL BELT-CINCHER...

Keep a calendar near your scale and record your weight everyday to monitor your progress and keep you motivated!!

*And Always Remember*:

**It's not what you can't have,
it's what you can have!**

# Author Acknowledgments

FOR THE LOVE, GENEROSITY AND support I received from my husband, Merle, family and friends, it is with heartfelt gratitude that I thank all who made this book possible.

I am deeply thankful that my friend and neighbor, Rosalie Castro, inspired me to write my grocery list and have it published, so that she could buy the list to give as gifts to her family and friends.

I am truly grateful for my friend Sharon McCarthy. I called her one day to ask what was new and exciting? She replied, "I lost 15 pounds in 15 weeks!" She is my inspiration and my support buddy who helped me start this book.

A special thanks to my Editor Helene Le Comte, a wonderful and talented Editor who transformed the manuscript and gave shape to my words, smoothing the structure, easing the flow, making the book much easier to read.

To my neighbor and author Kathy Verderber, for devoting countless hours helping to review, edit and shape volumes of information from the original manuscript. Your meticulous attention to detail, organization and input were invaluable in bringing this little book to life. You are truly amazing.

Special thanks to Jim Higgins, my I.P. Attorney, and Betty Higgins for inspiring me in the right path for success.

To Heather Donlan, a special thanks for my photo.

Special thanks to all at Balboa Press that have helped me create this Magical Grocery List ...*The Shrinking Belt*.

# Trademark Acknowledgments

The following companies listed below have given permission to share the products with my readers.

Bush's Best® Grillin' Beans® Black Bean Fiesta is a registered trademark of Bush Brothers & Company

Butter Buds® is a registered trademark of Cumberland Packing Corp., Brooklyn NY 11205

Cabot® Cabot Creamery

Campbell's® Healthy Request®, Campbell's® Select Harvest®, Franco-American®, Slow Roast®, and V8®Trademarks are used with permission of Campbell Soup Company"

Brother's International Food Corporation

Costco Wholesale Corporation

The Dannon Company, Inc.

Dreyer's/Edy's Grand Ice Cream

Finlandia Reduced Fat Cheese is the leading brand within the portfolio of Valio USA, a subsidiary of Valio LTD.

Flatout® Inc.

Francesco Rinaldi® and all associated logos and designs are registered trademarks of LiDestri Foods, Inc. and are used under license; To Be™ and To Be Healthy™ and all associated logos, designs and marks are trademarks of LiDestri Foods, Inc. and are used under license.

Fresh Gourmet® is a registered trademark of Sugar Foods Corporation and is used under license.

Hannah International Foods

Hodgson Mill Inc.

JOAN of ARC® is a registered trademark of B&G Foods, Inc. and/or its subsidiaries and is used under license."

JOLLY TIME® Pop Corn is a registered trademark of the American Pop Corn Company and is used under license."

Kahiki Foods, Inc.

Krusteaz® is a registered trademark of Continental Mills, Seattle, Washington USA

La Tortilla Factory is a registered trademark

Merita is a registered trademark of and used under license from Hostess Brands, Inc.

Mt. Olive Pickle Company, Inc.

NESTLÉ®, BUITONI®, CARNATION®, and LEAN CUSINE® are registered trademarks of Sociéte des Produits Nestlé S.A., Vevey, Switzerland. Used with permission.

Pepperidge Farm trademark used with permission of Pepperidge Farm, Incorporated

Polaner® a registered trademark of B&G Foods, Inc. and/or its subsidiaries and is used under license.

Post Cereals are used with permission from Post Foods, LLC.

Rosina Food Products, Inc.

Smart Balance® and Smart Beat® is a registered trademark of GFA Brands, Inc.

Snikiddy® is a registered trademark of Snikiddy, LLC

Seeds of Change® ©Mars, Incorporated

Shaw's Southern Belle Frozen Foods, Inc.

Trident Seafoods Corporation

Thomas is a registered trademark used with permission

Tam-x-icos® and Wrap-itz® are registered Trademarks owned by La Bonita Ole, Inc., Tampa, FL 33609

Van's Natural Foods™

Walden Farms, Inc., own registration for Walden Farms Calorie Free specialties

CPSIA information can be obtained at www.ICGtesting.com
Printed in the USA
BVOW04s0524111113

335979BV00005B/9/P